The Essentials of the Art of Medicine

An Essay Addressed to the Stillé Medical Society of the University of Pennsylvania.

By
Alfred Stillé, M.D., LL.D.

1897.

Theophania Publishing

THE ESSENTIAL ELEMENTS OF THE ART OF MEDICINE

"Factum præclarum atque divinum."—*Cicero.*

"Factis non annis vivunt mortales."
"Factis non verbis conditur medecina."
"Ars medica tota est in observationibus."
"Grau Freund ist alle Theorie,
Doch grün des Lebens goldener Baum."—*Goethe.*

THE search after truth has in every age been regarded as the most difficult, and often as the most fruitless of pursuits, for it has never been successful in revealing absolute truth, or that which is involved in and essential to any branch of knowledge. While it has demonstrated the honesty of some of the searchers and the perversity of others, it has resulted in the failure of all. Undoubtedly the cause of this failure has mainly been that no fact or proposition in natural science can be expressed in such precise terms as mathematicians use, and which, being abstract and clearly defined, are universally accepted at the same value in every age and place. But in the sciences of observation neither the facts nor their interpretation are definite, and the more complex a branch of knowledge is, the less uniform are the conclusions respecting it.

I leave out of this comparison the science of theology, the most anciently cultivated of all sciences, and which has always possessed the highest interest for the human mind. But since it relates to subjects which are in the province of faith rather than of reason, agreement in regard to it can never be reached by men who are free to judge and to act upon their judgments. It is far otherwise with natural and physical laws. Comparatively few are the differences of judgment among astronomers, but those which divide chemists and physicists are numerous; still more dissidents are to be met with among those who deal with living matter, with structure and function, normal and abnormal—that is to say, with physiology and pathology. But even their discordant opinions are slight compared with those that beset therapeutics.

Of it may be truly said that none of its principles are conclusively demonstrated, and that every alleged fact relating to it must be received only as a variable and fluctuating approach to truth; and if such is the case for those who have been, as far as may be, perfected in the science and art of medicine, much more emphatically is it so of the undergraduate. For him it is eminently true that "the aim of university teaching is not to perfect the student in knowledge, but to prepare him to learn." It is not absolute truth which men in general are competent to understand, nor is anyone competent to teach them; neither are they able duly to estimate those partial and approximate truths which even philosophers discern but dimly. Out of the multitude of devotees a few only are qualified to approach the sacred shrine. Even the most learned and gifted hardly do more than see it through a glass darkly. To the mass of mankind a faint and distant vision is alone possible. And even for them symbols of truth are provided in the formulæ of philosophy, and in the creeds and ceremonials of religion, which crudely overlie essential verities which even the acutest minds can but faintly behold and imperfectly comprehend.

In the remarks that are to follow I shall endeavor to illustrate the uncertainty of therapeutical laws, and show that it depends neither upon themselves, nor solely upon the fallibility of human judgment, but chiefly upon the extreme complexity and obscurity of the problems that occur in practical medicine. In that department of knowledge there is no constant quantity whatever, neither the physician, nor the patient, nor the remedy. The very complexity and uncertainty of clinical problems render the practice of medicine at once the most difficult and one of the most interesting of arts; interesting because its very purpose is the alleviation of suffering and the saving of life; difficult because its problems are the most complex the mind can examine; and uncertain because it concerns laws which, even as they relate to physical phenomena are very imperfectly known, while the relations of the mind to the body which it so powerfully affects can hardly be said to be known at all.

There was a period, and it lasted for centuries while the Galenical theories dominated the medical world, when the word of the Master drowned the voice of Nature. The falsely called science of mediæval times, which was too often as baseless as the clouds and as unstable as the sands of the desert, filled the schools with barren disputes and chimerical notions of the nature of diseases and their cures, and too often it was held to be more meritorious to be wrong with the Galen than to be right with nature.

An eminent man (De Tocqueville) has said that "in democracies general propositions are popular because they save the trouble of thinking." But their popularity is assuredly as great elsewhere, and for the same reason. In medicine they dispense physicians from that laborious research without which no substantial and lasting results can be reached. And when they are set forth with the fascinating art of speculative genius they draw around them a crowd of disciples who shrink from the slow and toilsome pursuit of the highest truth. So unsubstantial comets in their eccentric paths arouse more wonder than the stars, and the planets which move steadily and forever in their fixed orbits and give light and life to the universe. But during the dark ages in the history of medicine it must not be supposed that the darkness was complete; the night was illuminated by many stars that more or less guided minds strong enough to burst the shackles of conjectural systems, and which heralded the dawn that was ultimately to break upon every field of knowledge, and cause its hidden seeds to germinate and grow and bring forth fruit. Infinite pains and skill were needed to render its fruit palatable and nutritious—pains that no one man nor many generations could furnish, and which must be suffered to the very end of time. Every age, every generation, almost every period of a few years has witnessed greater or less changes in the doctrines, the principles, and the practice of medicine. If they are less ostensible and radical now than during the ages of inflexible theory and blind faith, if they come into view more gradually and gently, and grow distinct only through the lapse of time, it is because practical medicine is no longer so exclusively as it was the outcome of conjecture and speculation which reached their conclusions with a bound, but is rather a slow and vital growth of positive knowledge. The last resort in mooted questions is no longer authority which is individual and limited in power; appeal is made to the great Areopagus of learned and scientific men throughout the world. The word heretic (which really denotes no more than one who exercises his right of believing what he will—that is, the right of private judgment) is no longer the term of reproach and humiliation which for long ages it continued to be. Then it brought down the thunders of learned bodies, and blasted scientific free thinkers as effectually as did the fulminations of the Church the unhappy wretches who maintained their right to believe what their senses revealed to them and their reason approved. The days of persecution for opinion's sake seem to have passed away forever. The ridicule, discredit, and oppression that dogged the careers of Galileo, of Savonarola, of Harvey, of Jenner, and so many others whose names stand in the long martyrology of science, are hardly intelligible to the present generation, which has at least some reason to boast of its love of truth for truth's sake, and its freedom from prejudice. Yet it may well be questioned whether the charity and liberality that we claim for ourselves as virtues are not rather a result of the equality of civil rights in the modern world. It compels us to be tolerant of differences of opinion, to repress the invective that formerly was poured upon opponents, to conceal the claws which the animal in human nature too frequently incites us to employ against antagonists. It is a sad but unquestionable fact that the most virulent adversaries are men whose opinions and beliefs are least radically opposed. They are ready to grapple each other in deadly conflict over the meaning of some word, the significance of some fact, which neither understands, and yet will look with equanimity and even charity upon persons who agree with neither of them.

If liberty and equality under law effected nothing more than a compulsory deference, if not respect, for the habits, opinions, and even the prejudices of other men, they would justify their claim to the fetish-like worship they now command. It may be truly said of them that they refine men's manners and prevent their being brutal. But while there are limits within which differences of opinion should be courteously treated there is beyond them a region—"an abysmal valley dolorous" (*Inferno,* iv. 8)—filled with strange shapes, grotesque and vile, among which flit others shadowy and intangible. The former strive for recognition with brutal boldness; the latter with stealthy and insinuating manœuvres, and are apt to wheedle the self-sufficient rather than the ignorant into their snares. Upon the one the true physician looks with disgust, upon the other with contempt, striving meanwhile to keep his own skirts clear from the stains of similar coarseness or folly. He knows how great a heritage of knowledge and wisdom has come down to him through the ages, and strives to preserve it for his successors untainted by the defects and errors which it is impossible for any branch of knoweldge or any department of art to escape.

To this end it is important for him, and for us, to learn what are the boundaries of his field of knowledge, and what are the limits of his power within it. Above all, he should recognize the contrasts between medical science and medical art.

The science is limited strictly by a knowledge of structure and function. The limits of the art cannot be defined. In medical science (not mere theory) the facts are definite and do not readily admit of diverse interpretations. Once clearly determined, they are more or less fixed for all time. The history of medicine excites the wonder of every thoughtful student as he finds the descriptions of disease by Hippocrates or Aretœus, so far as they go, no less precise and accurate than those furnished by modern pathologists, because these physicians were content with picturing nature as they saw it. They remind one of the portraits recently discovered in the sepulchres of the Greek colonies in Egypt. Not heroic types such as poets described and sculptors represented, but real and familiar human countenances, with the same features and expressions that we constantly meet with in our daily walks. So, too, the features of diseases are essentially the same, whether pictured by Hippocrates or by the physicians of to-day. But in medical art the case is different. The facts and laws of practical therapeutics are unstable, and their interpretation is uncertain. In this as in every other department of knowledge, ignorance and vanity are active and aggressive in the direct proportion of the intricacy and obscurity of the subject discussed. In the domains of anatomy (normal or morbid) and in physiology the passions have little opportunity to exhibit themselves, because in these sciences rigorous laws rebuke and repel pretenders whose ignorance soon brings them into contempt. But in therapeutics there is no one, from the learned and ingenious spinner of theories to the ignorant and credulous dispenser of nostrums—often absurd or disgusting—who does not assume for himself a mental penetration which accomplished therapeutists modestly but emphatically disclaim. If there is any branch of knowledge in which modesty and humility are becoming it is that which concerns the action of medicines and their curative powers, for in them the elements are infinite in number and constant in their inconstancy. How cautious should we be in formulating laws in this branch of medicine when we remember that the strictest rules of interpretation have been applied only in the most exact of all natural sciences—astronomy. Yet it is related that Newton was asked one day what enabled him to walk as he willed, and he boldly answered, "I do not know." But, said the inquirer, surely you who are so familiar with the laws of gravitation can explain to me why the earth and all the planets revolve only in one direction; but again he answered, "I do not know." As in Newton's case, so in our own, it will often be a mark of wisdom to confess ignorance, just as it is too often the sign of an ignorant, pretentious man to profess a knowledge of things he does not understand. Judged by this test, how few scientific physicians could justify their claim to wisdom; for they are addicted to explaining everything, and, unlike Newton, feel so humiliated by admitting their ignorance, that they are apt to offer vague or even impossible or unintelligible explanations rather than confess that they do not know.

The dawn of recorded medical history is distinguished by two contrasting characters—positiveness in the description of diseases, and doubt, reserve, and simplicity in their treatment. Later on, and in proportion as medicine drifted away from the simple and natural Hippocratic standards, to be engulfed in the turbid waters of the Galenical system and the other systems of which it was the prolific parent, the clinical aspects of medicine were hidden by the clouds of theory and system-building. Even at the present day the medical profession has not recovered from the effects of this error, and nothing is more common in medical books and periodicals than to meet with the statement that certain therapeutical measures are "indicated" by the assumed nature of the disease, when it should merely be declared that experience had or had not justified their use. "The natural tendency to reckon words as equivalent to facts, and assertions to demonstrations, always gives (theologians) theorists and (metaphysicians) speculators, an immense advantage over observers" (Nordau, *Degeneration,* p. 76). It seems to be forgotten that the nature of diseases is often suggested, and even determined, by the action upon them of the remedies employed in their treatment, whether by aggravating their symptoms or moderating them, or by lessening or prolonging the duration of the attack. It is not enough because a disease belongs to the class of inflammations that it should be treated antiphlogistically; nor is it true that the typhoid type always calls for stimulants; nor that narcotics are indispensable when ataxic or nervous phenomena predominate, or even when pain occurs.

In medical as in social science, it is certain that general laws deduced from the nature of things, or even arrived at through inductive reasoning, or any other general logical process, are seldom, if ever, applicable to the solution of questions concerning individuals alone. All generalization of facts, or general propositions resting on facts, and which are denominated laws, are formed by the aggregation of those things in which the facts are similar; but they for that very reason leave out of sight these elements which are dissimilar, incongruous, or even hostile or incompatible, and which, therefore, cannot be classed together or referred to any single law, scientific or empirical. This statement is true of every department of knowledge. It is notoriously true of political economy, whose principles are viewed in contrasted lights by the political parties which divide communities and even nations; it is also true of civil and criminal law, whose fundamental principles are accepted by all civilized peoples, but which in practice are not applied by any two alike; it is true even of moral science, whose foundations of right and wrong are recognized by all nations and in every age, but whose practical applications are as various as the communities that adopt them for their government; it is also true of every one of the arts of which scientific principles form the rational basis. Every particular instance requires a greater or less modification of the general principles involved in it. "Inventors, great and small, are rarely theorists; the invention must, before all things, be suited to the necessity, and the theory may come afterward if anybody cares for it. For a theory is nothing but an attempted explanation, and the fact must exist before it can possibly need explaining. Bread is a great invention against hunger, and a man needs to know nothing about gastric juices to save himself from starvation when the loaf is at hand" (M. Crawford). Political economists have never made successful statesmen; the most learned judges are far from being the best forensic lawyers; the profoundest analysts of moral motives are not always the most incorruptible and upright men; no acquaintance with the theory of colors will make a painter famous; no knowledge of the structure of language will make a poet or an orator; none of mechanics will create an accomplished engineer; and no familiarity with anatomy, etiology, pathology, or therapeutics and materia medica will of itself render a physician skilful in diagnosis and successful in the treatment of disease. To this end must be added the one thing needful, personal fitness, sagacity in recognizing the peculiarities of individual cases, and in adapting the treatment of them, hygienic, dietetic, and medicinal, to the special requirements of each. In a word, the physician must never forget that he has a patient as well as a disease to treat. It may be objected that attainments of such a judicial character as I have suggested are seldom to be met with in history or in one's own experience. That is very true; but it is no reason for rejecting a model that one cannot imitate it perfectly. The medical, like all other professions, is made up of very diverse and unequal members, and yet when we consider it as a whole, and at the proper distance of time and space, we find that these irregularities diminish or disappear. Did you ever witness an eclipse of the moon and observe the perfectly even outline of the earth's shadow upon its satellite? Not the slightest irregularity is visible. Our Himalayas, and Alps, and Andes, the gigantic peaks which stud the eastern and western continents, cast no shadow there. And so it is with human achievements when we study them from a point of vantage. The mighty men of valor and the puny dwarfs, the philosophers and the fools, the law-givers and the men of renown for all that makes illustrious figures in history—they all shrink down to a common level in the earth from which they sprang, and to which they must sooner or later return again.

Properly considered, medical education is a branch of general education. Its true foundations are in general science, philosophy, and literature. It must, like other edifices, be built up by adding stone to stone, course to course, story to story. A house cannot be built in the air, nor can we create a science or an art unless it rests upon foundations consolidated by time and approved by experience. In vain do we try to detach it from its origin and its history. As well might we expect a tree to bring forth fruit if we uproot it from the ground out of which it sprang. Attempts have never ceased to claim for it an independent existence. But, as I have said, we cannot build a house in the air. We may try to suspend medicine by the balloons of theory, and the vulgar may applaud our ingenious inventions, but sooner or later the gas escapes from them, and the baseless fabric rushes to the ground.

It has been said that every nation in the long run possesses the best government it is fitted for. And it is at least equally true that the social and intellectual condition of a nation represents the best it is at the time fitted to enjoy. It is impossible to create at a stroke, as if by an enchanter's wand, a civilized nation out of barbarous tribes, or without due time for growth; to develop a literary, scientific, or polished society among a people who are struggling to overcome the obstacles set up by nature, and the crude ideas, language, and habits which these material hindrances beget. It is not disgraceful for a nation to be merely ignorant of literature, science, or art; but it is a reproach to any people to remain obstinately attached to its ignorance and errors.

There was a time, and that quite within the memory of the elders of our profession, when physicians of reputation, and who even filled official positions as teachers in medical schools, were not ashamed to promulgate such doctrines, and actively and even zealously oppose every hint and resent every declaration which implied that the teaching of medicine in this country was disgracefully crude and narrow. They stigmatized those who clamored for a nearer assimilation of our schools and of the profession to the best models of the old world as unpatriotic, if not disloyal. We may be thankful that the awakened spirit of the age overcame these encumberers and obstructionists, and relegated them to the dark regions where the murkier atmosphere was better fitted to their undeveloped faculties. The medical profession at that time underwent a notable development, but chiefly through the ever-growing numbers and influence of those who spent more or less time in European schools. Through them light flamed out in every direction to illuminate the dark places of American medicine until it became possible for American physicians to feel a well-founded pride in the progress of their profession.

As I survey the vast field where at the present day so many accomplished laborers are constantly enriching us with harvests of scientific and practical knowledge, I am obliged to recall the meeting of the Medical Congress held in this city in 1876. I had the honor of presiding in the Section on Practical

Medicine. Many of the speakers were eminent physicians from various parts of Europe, and one could not fail to admire and even envy their erudition and their scientific and practical knowledge, and the moderation and clearness of their language. These qualities were all the more striking when contrasted with the barren, illogical, and flimsy addresses of too many of our countrymen who seemed far better qualified for haranguing political mobs than taking part in the grave discussions of scientific and remedial questions in medicine. So mortifying an experience I had never before endured, and I think it could hardly befall one now, so largely has the vain dream been dispelled which long was cherished that America was competent to create an exclusively American science and art of medicine, and which tended to hold back the wheels of medical progress. No one doubts at present that medicine had its roots in the very dawn of humanity, and has never ceased to grow in stature and strength, and by its very nature must continue to grow while mankind survives and disease and injuries occur.

I cannot quite end this digression without first prolonging it to illustrate the difference between teaching and professing to teach. It was said of an eminent professor in the University of Oxford that "he had what may be described as the tutorial character, but not the professorial mind." The former of these terms appears to me a suitable description of the teaching which was long in vogue, and is probably extant still in some of our medical schools. It took its rise in the day of small things, but clings tenaciously to some of them still. Until within the last generation not a few professors degraded their teaching to the level of a dame's school by prefacing every lecture with an examination on the previous one. And then the professorial body was not entirely without those anencephalous creatures who year after year rehearsed the same lectures without note, emendation, or addition; who never added anything to the science or art of medicine, but continued rehearsing their parrot cry until the end. Little they recked of the student's thirst for knowledge, and as little seemed conscious that medicine was perpetually changing as a science and as an art. If the professor slumbers the student cannot remain awake, unless it be to resent as dishonest that he should be given a stone instead of the bread that he asked for and paid for. Such a professor was not likely to stimulate the student's mind, to make him think, observe, classify, and analyze his observations; for he was not apt to create in his pupils a craving for what he did not himself possess. His method was distinctly tutorial and not professorial. He alone is a competent professor who can claim at the end of his career that of all his pupils he has been the one most profited by his labors. The greatest men in the ranks of science or literature have been, not the tutors who dealt exclusively in second-hand thoughts, but professors who either originated what was new, or so treated what was not new, as to give it a novel charm and a new efficiency, and while doing so interested their pupils as to make their study a labor of love. From this excursion into the ethical region of my subject I return to the starting point.

It was long ago declared that the art of medicine is founded wholly on the observation of disease. But in all observation there are two factors—the observer and the observed. The thing observed is constant and unchangeable under identical conditions; but observers are perpetually changing and liable to change. So that, although the thing or fact may remain the same the accounts of it given by different observers, or by the same observer under varying conditions, may differ widely from each other, according as the object is seen under different lights, under different angles of vision, in different associations. Or the observer may perceive it differently, owing to nearsightedness, or color-blindness, or the medium through which it is examined, or even because he has preconceived— that is, prejudiced— opinions of what its appearance ought to be. In short, the judgments we form of things external to us, and even of our internal perceptions, are not invariable nor consistent with one another. They are made up of external realities and internal impressions and conceptions. Color-blindness may be mentioned as a familiar illustration of the errors into which our senses may lead us. It often happens that one cannot distinguish the color of ripened fruit from that of the leaves around it. And certain artist painters who excelled in drawing and composition, owing to color-blindness have produced pictures that were caricatures of nature. The examination of railroad signal-men has showed that this strange defect is not uncommon. But there is also a mental, and there is a moral "colorblindness" which seems to pervert the judgment and the conscience; the good and the true of one person may be the evil and the false of another. Whether this defect be inherited or is the outcome of a vicious education, it lies at the root of the greater number of the differences that divide mankind into nations, and nations into political, and religious, and scientific, and artistic sects. Most of all does it, perhaps, exist in those branches of knowledge which contain a mixture of facts and speculations, and in which, even when the facts are themselves demonstrable, their relations among themselves and to other facts are apt to be differently perceived and estimated by different persons.

It follows, then, that a perfect consensus of opinion upon any subject that is not abstractly or mathematically demonstrable, or that is not imposed by authority, is not to be looked for, and that the most favorable result, as regards practical as well as speculative knowledge, is an enlightened and candid and eager search for truth, a search conducted with all the light furnished by history and experience, with a steadfast adherence and devotion to truth; and, when truth has been found, a stern refusal to be seduced from allegiance to it by any ardent appeal or any plausible arguments offered in the name of liberalism, or any subtle temptations to propose or accept compromises, in the name of uprightness and truth, but really for the promotion of selfish interests.

In addition to all these hindrances to a search for medical and for other truths is the notorious fact that medical literature is full of the products of ignorance, unskilfulness, and even deceit, and hence that the simple truth seldom stands out clearly. The half-educated and the inexperienced observer or commentator is very apt to deceive others while he deceives himself. What he does not discern clearly he cannot make clear to others. A very significant phrase is attributed to Carlyle, to the effect that a teacher or writer "should learn to consume his own smoke." In this remark allusion was made to the noisy puffing of dark smoke by a steam engine before it begins its most efficient work; or, perhaps, to the ordinary chimney fire, that before it burns with a clear, glowing flame, sends forth volumes of smoke that fills the air and clogs the chimney. The simile is an apt one applied to inventors in mechanics, art, literature, or science, and especially to the young and inexperienced among them. In their eagerness to win fame they are tempted to parade their productions before a critical world and then, if their work is neglected or condemned, they are apt to feel surprise and, perhaps, resentment that the world failed to see their fire through the smoke they raised. But Carlyle's homely metaphor is only a variant of the Horation maxim *Prematur in nonum.* A nine years' gestation is often as necessary for a literary work as nine months are for a human progeny. It never deserved to be pondered more carefully than at the present day, when every fledgling in science or literature feels impelled to spread his wings for a flight toward the stars, too often forgetful of the melancholy fate of Icarus. But not only does immaturity of intellect produce abortions in science and art, but it also generates many that are feeble and incoherent rather than incomplete. A saying attributed to Napoleon is that

"A general should indulge in no mental pictures, but look at things clearly, as through a field-glass," and this thought may be applied to observation in general. Concentration of attention is, first of all, essential to accuracy of vision; for if the thing observed is not clearly discerned its relation to other objects cannot be determined. So in natural science and in art the mind must, first of all, distinctly apprehend the thing that is to be studied, and after that its relation to associated things. So in medicine the only safe clue to an accurate conception of disease is through a minute study of all its forms and relations and the modifications they undergo through internal and external influences, and, next to those the variations imposed upon them by hygienic and therapeutic measures, *i. e.*, by treatment.

We hear a great deal of "the advance of medicine," and are often reminded of discoveries made in human and comparative anatomy and physiology through vivisection, experimental phyisiology, and chemistry, and are apt to believe that before us all the world was in darkness. But if the light of the present day does not dazzle us so much as to prevent our reading the history of medicine aright, we shall be surprised at the uniformity of the pictures of disease bequeathed to us by ancient writers, and of their identity with those that nature furnishes us to-day. It is not the diseases, but the theories invented to explain them, that have undergone the greatest mutations. These and the medicines employed to cure them have varied as continually as the dogmas that were used to explain the one and the other. Thus it came to pass that, as I have already suggested, medical art has always been unstable, while the facts that form the basis of medical science have remained essentially unchanged.

In medicine, as in every other department of knowledge that is founded upon a study and correlation of natural phenomena, this double quality exists—a substratum of positive, demonstrable, and imperishable truth, and a superstructure of more artificial and transient materials imposed by the instinctive longing of the mind for explanations and laws, and, in default of substantial principles, for theories however crude and hypotheses however wild. Theories in the natural sciences are no more essential to them than the clothing we wear is essential to our structure and functions; but we have come so thoroughly to identify men by their garb that we should scarcely recognize them in a nude condition. And so we are prone to confound the substantial facts of pathology and therapeutics with the theories that envelop them and claim to represent them. This blindness to the true nature and aims of science and art is a serious impediment to our acquiring a just conception of either. What has been said of another department of knowledge is equally true of medicine: "The scientific writer should confine himself to describing and picturing what he sees, without attempting to frame any theory, even in the innermost recesses of his mind. Without this precaution the most careful observer is liable to become a dupe of 'expectant attention,' and to see things in accord with his preconceived notions rather than with the facts" (*The Nation,* January 15, 1896, p. 107). There is a wide difference between facts and formulas. Yet there are many young physicians, as well as callow students, who feel able to tell you all about the work done by every organ of the body; how the chyle is converted into blood, and the blood into living tissue, indeed, into a score of tissues all elaborated from the same identical fluid which seems so homogeneous; they can explain to you how this nerve is the organ of sensation, and that of motion, and how a third marshalls in one army the various corps that perform this or that function—they can unravel a multitude of such mysteries with as much (or as little) real knowledge, and yet you may search in vain for one who can demonstrate the nature of diseases, and still less their cure. There is no formula by which you may cure consumption, or pneumonia, or a specific fever, or any other disease under the sun. The student or young physician who has felt so sure of himself while he was expounding the mysteries of physiology, stands silent and abashed before the rationale of the simplest therapeutic act; and so little is he sure of the remedies he should choose that after he has expended all his laboratory science, and even all his skill derived from experience upon an apparently simple question, he is obliged to confess that vital problems are too deep for him to understand, and that his highest real achievement in therapeutics must be the employment of not the most certain remedies, but the best authenticated by reason and experience, and so feel entitled to hope for, but never to be absolutely sure of, the desired result.

An eminent man of science has emphasized his condemnation of the popular notions upon this subject by saying that "An *explanation* is never given by science: the whole of science is *description*" (Prof. Karl Pearson, *Fortnightly Review,* November, 1895, p. 675). The interpretation of the things described may, and indeed must, vary more or less with the mental nature and the competency of the interpreter. And so the less of one's self one weaves into the descriptions he gives of diseases and of their treatment, the more faithfully will he represent the truth of nature, and the nearer will he approach a likeness to those great physicians who, from Hippocrates to our own day, have "held the mirror up to nature."

What has been said of one of the greatest thinkers of modern times, Goëthe, may serve as the pattern of all natural philosophers, and especially of rational physicians: "He possessed the patient observation, the reliance on careful experiment, the aversion to hasty theorizing, the instinct for so co-ordinating numerous facts into a general law which collectively mark the highest scientific genius" (John Owen, *The Five Great Sceptical Dramas,* p. 220).

But clinical, experimental, and, indeed, every form of observation is intended not only to preserve a photographic picture of bare facts, but also to produce a special grouping and sequence of facts that will demonstrate their natural and logical interdependence and their relation to the end or purpose for which their investigation is made. It is the power of doing this that distinguishes the handicraftsman in medicine, and in every art, from the true artist, and enables its possessor to demonstrate what is proper and essential to the subject or thing investigated, and raises him above the mere clerk who records, or the photographer who imitates, and assimilates him to the author who inspires and the artist who creates. This faculty, which has been called the scientific imagination, is not the faculty of the poet, by which he sees things that do not really exist, but the power of mentally conceiving or realizing the whole of a picture of which a part only is presented to the senses. It is this scientific imagination which derives its value from the uniformity of nature, and enables one not to speculate at random under the spur of the imagination, but by obeying the laws of cause and effect, and the associations which nature infallibly creates, to become a faithful intepreter of nature's laws. It is this faculty which essentially distinguishes the philosopher from the poet, and enables one to follow a straight path on the firm earth, while the poet on the wings of his imagination soars beyond the verge of human reason.

I venture once more to repeat my lifelong declaration of faith that every art must exist before its associated science, and that, how much soever each may illustrate the other, both are essentially independent. Neither botany, nor chemistry, nor pharmacy, nor pharmaco-dynamics, nor physiology, nor bacteriology, is an essential part of therapeutics. Its true and only foundation is clinical medicine, the medicine which recognizes and treats diseases. Medicine, in this sense, is an art and not a science; its laws are rules established, not by theory, but by observation and experience. They are as various as the medicines employed or as the patients who take them; they must be modified by the nature, the form, the tendencies of the particular disease, by the external and the internal conditions and relations of the patients. The certainty of a science depends upon the fixity or constancy of its elements; the uncertainty of the healing art is due to the inconstancy, the fluctuating values of the elements involved in the disease, in the remedies, in the patient, and in the physician himself, elements which no science has ever measured or reduced to law, and which none probably ever will; but what science has failed to do for disease in general, and for classes of diseases, practical sagacity has accomplished for indvidual patients.

There is a science, and there is an art, of medicine, but the boundary line between them is not always clearly defined: for although we may arbitrarily separate the one from the other, it is evident that while both are independent in their nature, each tends to throw light upon the other—the science upon the art, by enabling us to group together empirical facts in an order and arrangement which makes both the science and the art more intelligible; and the art upon the science, by providing it with a wider basis of facts for induction, and by tending through clinical experience to rectify the errors inseparable from the application of normal to abnormal laws. The familiar anecdote, whether it be literally true or not, which relates that the law of gravitation was revealed to Newton by the fall of an apple, or that other equally striking story that the oscillation of a chandelier suggested to Galileo the orbit of the planets, serves to show that in the portion of the domain of knowledge, where the laws are unchangeable, a sagacious mind may leap from a single fact to a boundless generalization. But this rapid and intuitive faculty is always inborn, one of those mental operations that we attribute to genius, and which is unknown to the average mind. It is like the power to declare the result of arithmetical calculations more rapidly than they can be worked out by the most expert accountant. No calculating prodigy has ever been able to describe the process by which such astonishing results are reached; and, strange to say, these natural arithmeticians have generally been otherwise quite undistinguished either as mathematicians or in the common business of life. Sometimes, indeed, they have ceased to possess their phenomenal faculty on attaining adult age. In practical affairs, and conspicuously in practical medicine, this instinctive faculty is apt to be designated as common sense, and, when habitually exercised upon concrete facts, and not upon abstract numbers, is rendered stronger and more manageable by time and exercise, and those who possess it are looked up to as wise men in their several spheres, and are appealed to in doubtful cases. They possess an authority which they have derived not from science alone, nor from experience alone. Not infrequently they give wise and just opinions, the reasons for which they are unable satisfactorily to state. Their faculty is innate, however it may be perfected by use, just as the surgeon's hand, however adroit by nature, grows incomparably more so by practice. The talent for acquiring languages, which is so conspicuous in a few rare and phenomenal cases, was carried to an extreme limit in the case of Cardinal Mezzofanti, who is reported to have spoken one hundred languages. Yet of the structure of them he was entirely ignorant, and he was unable to teach them. Still more striking, and yet more common, are the instances of musical prodigies, and of poets, "who lisped in numbers" almost from infancy; of mechanicians also who even in childhood showed a genius for invention which afterward made them famous.

In like manner there are physicians by instinct as well as by education; just as there are many persons whom the most assiduous training can never make great linguists, musicians, artists, or scientists, so are there not a few whom all the learning, and science of the schools and all the bedside training of the hopitals, indeed, all the experience of a lifetime can never transform into skilful, wise, and prudent physicians. It has been well said that "the men called great who have risen to distinction are not men of brains but of aptitude." Among physicians nature has granted them the gift of insight by which to discern the essential elements of individual diseases, as well as those which they have in common with other diseases, and to weigh their value in special cases; and also the co-ordinate talent for selecting the fittest medicines and duly adjusting their doses, combinations, and times and modes of administration. An old Scotch doctor is said to have remarked of one of his young competitors in practice: "He's one of the kind they turn out in plenty nowadays: all theory and no grit." And by "grit" he meant those minute particulars I have just enumerated, and upon which the efficacy of medicines so largely depends. It should never be forgotten that the patient has no direct concern with the learning and science of his physician, and is incapable of estimating their value. They are of interest to him in so far only as they are reinforced by the physician's tact in seizing the essential elements of his patient's disease, and his dexterity in adapting his remedies, not so much to the nominal affection, as to the actual, living, suffering, endangered patient before him. After all that science and experience can teach him, he may still lack the essential faculty which is the power to see, and know, and judge the condition of his patient, not only in its entirety, but in every individual element.

This power, or tact, is a peculiar faculty. It resembles instinct, for it reaches a definite object without a consciousness of the intervening steps. On the other hand, it is allied to the imagination, for it leaps from premises to conclusions in disregard of those steps if, indeed, it is conscious of them. To an exceptional few the relations of the two ends of the chain are revealed in a flash, as it were, of that divine fire which we call genius. By the greater number the relations are discovered by long, laborious, and repeatedly fruitless experiment. The conclusions of the former we call brilliant, and they really are so in their meteoric rapidity and brightness; but their duration is apt to be brief and their utility is questionable. The results of slower, more deliberate and searching methods are more frequently substantial and permanent. Undoubtedly the most reliable physician is one who combines in due proportion the illumination of genius and a calm, judicial analysis and estimate of the case he is called upon to treat.

His power is most surely exhibited by that supreme tact which enables him to eliminate from a case its non-essential elements and wisely adapt his remedies to those which make up, as it were, the body of the disease, and upon which its issue practically depends. To accomplish this purpose he will, first of all, determine whether his active interference with the evolution of the disease is necessary or will be advantageous. He is the spectator of a combat between nature and disease, and knows that it must be "fought to a finish." He knows that, whether assisted or not, nature will determine the issue of the conflict, and it is only when nature falters or fails that the physician should interfere to sustain her and put down her enemy. He should withhold his armament of drugs unless the necessity of using it becomes imperative, and be content rather to remove hindrances out of nature's way than to employ his drugs as her substitute. It is too frequently forgotten that we run great risk of resisting the restorative powers of nature when we attempt to substitute for them agencies of our own devising. Even when we employ them it is wise to use them gently, lest we injure where we intended to help. We should remember the ancient fable of the bear that in his attempt to drive the flies from his master's face crushed it to a jelly. Whatever else of his studies the educated physician may forget, he should always remember the *ne quid nimis* of the ancients, and learn that by holding and using too many weapons at once he runs the risk of using none efficiently.

Two hundred years ago Sir William Temple, one of the most sagacious, learned, and experienced men of his time, in a discourse upon the gout, from which he had suffered, as well as from many things of many physicans, wrote as follows (*Works,* iii. 248): "I had passed twenty years of my life and several accidents of danger in my health without any use of physicians; and from some experiments of my own as well as much reading and thought upon that subject, had reasoned myself into the opinion that the use of them and their methods (unless in some sudden and acute diseases) was itself a very great venture, and that their greatest practisers practised least upon themselves or their friends. *I have even quarrelled with their studying art more than nature, and applying themselves to methods rather than remedies, whereas the knowledge of the last is all that nine parts in ten of the world have been trusted to in all ages.*"

If one reads reflectively the professional literature of the present day he will be apt to be a good deal of Sir William Temple's opinion. He can hardly fail of being surprised at the complacency of medical writers to whom their science seems to present no mysteries, and their art no difficulties, so glibly do they expound riddles that have perplexed the wise in preceding ages, and so jauntily do they make light of the nature and cure of diseases which have always defied the maturest skill and which continue to resist the most consummate art, notwithstanding the loud promises and positive assertions of physicians who are too often ignorant of medical history and of the conditions of cure taught by personal experience. They make but little account of that quintessence of wisdom which Hippocrates at the first distilled, and which has come down to us through the ages unimpaired, and is as true to-day as when it was uttered twenty-four centuries ago: "Life is short but Art is long, and the opportunities of learning it are fleeting; for things are often not what they seem, and to judge them is difficult." How solemnly true does this oracular judgment seem to those who have learned the hollowness of the vauntings of science and art which float down the stream of Time as a part of the rubbish that is swept into the ocean of forgetfulness.

An English writer lamenting the deterioration of domestic economy in his own country, which once was famous for the good order, cleanliness, and happiness of its homes, attributes it to the erroneous education of the young, who are crammed with all manner of useless knowledge and at the same time are allowed to remain ignorant of, or unskilled in, the things that make wholesome and happy homes while fitting them to earn their bread by superor skill in definite occupations. "There has been," he says, "enough of mere instruction; and our people are fast sinking into cultivated impotence" (*London Quarterly,* July, 1895, p. 70). Have we no reason to apply this judgment to ourselves? Have we not, in our eagerness to cultivate the science of medicine been guilty of decrying and neglecting medical art? There was a time when either medical schools did not exist or were held to be secondary to personal and practical instruction. There was also a time which, indeed, continued almost to the present day, when the medical student was an apprenticed pupil for a term of years, during which he performed such almost menial services as his preceptor required. Little he recked of the sciences of etiology, pathology, or pharmaco-dynamics, yet he learned how to recognize diseases, their phases and tendencies, and the remedies appropriate for their cure. He was profoundly ignorant ofmicrobean pathology and experimental therapeutics. If he happened to be judicious and sagacious and capable of recognizing the truth, he did not shrink from confessing that in a large class of cases nature is the sole curer of disease (*Medicus curat, Natura sanat, morbos*), and that to her and not to the apothecary, should be confided substantially the treatment of the sick.

Surely at the present day we are scarcely warranted in resenting the imputation that much learning hath made us mad. At the bedside of the sick, where the issues of life and death are often in our hands, we are too apt to turn for guidance to the positive assurances of the laboratory and the torture-room of the physiologist, rather than listen to the still, small, voice that whispers the suggestions of wisdom and experience. The dogmatic assurances of science may be consolatory to the discomfited intelligence, but they are merely anodynes, not cures, for the baneful errors into which they have allured us. We turn from them disappointed, but confirmed in our conviction that when a medicine cures a disease or relieves a symptom, it matters very little whether or not we comprehend the manner in which its effect is produced. Must I once more repeat what I have never ceased to insist upon: that the most positive and certain effects of medicines are precisely those we are least able to explain. Do we know how opium or any other narcotic or anæsthetic produces sleep or relieves pain? Or how mercury cures syphilis? Or iodine removes goitre? How arsenic is a remedy for intermittent fever, and also for skin diseases and neuralgia? How quinine cures as well as prevents periodical fevers and periodical neuralgia? How the bromides suspend epilepsy or the salicylates rheumatism? And yet these are familiar and daily examples. No; we know nothing of their mode of cure, and to mask and cloak our ignorance we call it *specific!* What then are the proper guides in medical therapeutics? First undoubtedly is the determination of the disease or condition which is to be treated. Next to this, and of hardly less importance, are the conditions under which the disease arises, its special type and its external circumstances. Of these some are external, as climate, season, weather. Others are individual, as sex, age, constitution, habits, idiosyncracies, and susceptibilities. It is very true that "it is appointed unto all men once to die," or, as the Latin poet tells us,

"Pallida mors æquo pede pulsat

Regum que turres et pauperum tabernas."

Ghastly death, with an impartial step, knocks at the palace gate and at the pauper's door. But before death's advent there may be, and usually are, many occasions in which the physician's skill prevents the fatal visit, and his power is never more conspicuous than when its exercise is modified by the nativity, the social rank, the habits and other conditions of the patient. He knows that the coarse and callous fibre of men whose daily bread depends upon their daily toil in the open air, exposed to all the vicissitudes of the weather, may tolerate, and, indeed, require heroic measures that might be fatal to persons nursed in the lap of luxury and whose systems respond intensely to slight impressions and tend to sink under an enfeebling medication. For this reason it is that the physician who is chiefly trained in hospitals finds, when he enters the luxurious chambers of the rich, that the methods he once considered gentle are quite unsuited to his present *clientele*, with whom even the mildest medicinal measures must often be supplemented by a tonic or soothing regimen addressed not only to the malady but also to the mental and moral nature.

Even from this passing glance at the conditions that must modify every plan of treatment, it is evident that to assert of a particular medicine or method that it is the most efficient in a given disease is to convey very little information. It furnishes, as it were, only the skeleton of a therapeusis which we are called on to clothe with living flesh and endow with living organs before we can learn how to employ it profitably. Hence, without illustrating the subject further, it seems evident that all the science one may possess can furnish him with nothing more than a bare foundation on which to build the treatment of individual cases. All cases are complex, no two are precisely alike in their pathological elements, no two patients are identical in their susceptibilities and tendencies, or in the manner and degree in which medicines affect them. The least clinical experience will satisfy an observant physician that pneumonia, for instance, which is so demonstrable a disease, and in most cases has so definite a history, yet runs very different courses in its several forms, which may be asthenic or typhoid, simple, complicated, bilious, malarial, etc., and that to propose a fixed method of treatment for pneumonia is simply preposterous. Similar remarks are applicable to typhus fever, typhoid fever, to the eruptive fevers, rheumatism, neuralgia, and many other affections. So that while there ought to be a certain scheme, or model plan of treatment for all cases of a disease included under a common name, that standard must be susceptible of modification, even to complete reversal, if the varying conditions of the case demand it. In other words, the sagacity of the physician must be so great, and his attention so constantly on the alert, as to bend his method in any direction required by the exigencies of the moment. There may be a fitting place for the discussion of theories in the class-room of the lecturer or in the medical society, but there is also one place where they should rarely be allowed to intrude, and that is at the bedside of the sick. Health and life are very precious, and are too precarious at the best to be rendered more so by the vagaries of medical speculation.

A critical writer has blamed the custom of historians who treat of every country as an independent entity, and refer all its advancing and retrograde movements in the march of civilization to the peculiar qualities of its own inhabitants, whereas it is certain that every State has been influenced and modified by the conditions of the States around it and its relations with them. So that it is only in a general way that a particular people can be said to possess certain national characteristics. The same truth applies to many analogous subjects, none of which can be strictly defined, and whose tendencies and issues cannot be unerringly anticipated. It is eminently so with the subjects that concern us as practical physicians. The wider, the more scientific our generalizations are the further they depart from the truth as it is in nature, which is concerned not at all with generalizations, but with individual facts. What they gain in breadth they loose in strength and truth. The more particulars a definition embraces (of any organic class, from man down to the humblest zoophyte), the less accurately does it describe any individual of the series. No vital phenomenon, no remedial agency, presents twice in succession precisely the same proportions, relations, degrees, and results. Out of all the experience gathered by ourselves or others we may construct an ideal disease or plan of treatment, but the very next case of that disease we encounter may diverge more or less widely from our ideal conception of it, and we may find that the methods of treatment on which we have heretofore relied with confidence require material modification. Herein the laws of life differ widely from the laws of dead matter. Herein medical science diverges most from medical art in which a wise and clinically taught practitioner becomes more valuable to his patients and to the community than the most accomplished pathologist or the most consummate adept in experimental therapeutics. Our art is personal and individual in its application; and, however wide the field from which we may derive our knowledge and our skill in exercising it, we can never employ aright its vast resources unless we are able to gather them all together and apply them not only to a particular form of fever, inflammation, or degeneration, but also, and above all, adapt them to the individual man, woman, or child for whom we exercise the office of a physician.

Let me further illustrate the relations between the science and the art of medicine. However we may explain it or attempt to justify it, there can be no doubt that in all ages and nations, in Eastern lands, in Egypt and Greece, and in the countries that inherited their knowledge, there have always been two classes in the community—one that governed and one that obeyed; one that knew and one that only believed; one acquainted with the laws of nature, the other only familiar with their practical effects; one governed by princples, the other by the letter of the laws; one forever striving after a knowledge of causes, the other as constantly concerned with particular facts alone. Thus there was and is a science of religion to which no single form of religious belief or ceremonial every conformed; a science of law which is far from being practically regarded as much as precedents and statutes are; and a science of medicine which has as little direct application to the art of healing as creeds have to morality or the administration of laws to the principles of jurisprudence. There may be morality under pagan faiths as there is crime and licentiousness under the most elevated religious beliefs; and there were wise, skilful, and successful therapeutists before the discovery of the circulation of the blood, or of the structure or functions of the nervous system, or any accurate knowledge of the functions of a single organ had been acquired. I said a moment ago that there were successful therapeutists before the discovery of the circulation of the blood, and I venture to emphasize the statement that this supreme anatomical and physiological fact has had little direct bearing upon the healing art. In a letter of Thomas Jefferson is stated what appears to me the truth upon this point, in the following words: "Harvey's discovery of the circulation of the blood was a beautiful addition to our knowledge of the ancient economy; but on a review of the practice of medicine before and since that epoch, I do not see any great amelioration which has been derived from that discovery" (*Medical News,* lxviii. 731). We should be very careful to distinguish between our knowledge of phenomena and our interpretations of them. The knowledge may be more or less imperfect, but so far as it is accurate it is also true; but with rare exceptions our rationale or theory of the laws of those phenomena is inaccurate, is never complete, and is always provisional.

Of therapeutics we may say what has been said of the legislative powers in a State. We cannot assign definite and immutable limits to them, or lay down inflexible rules for their use. The treatment of every case of sickness must be determined ultimately for and by itself, tentatively by skilled men, and as their practical sagacity may determine, while they bear in mind that the virtues of a medicine depend less upon its intrinsic properties and powers than on the sagacity of the physician who administers it; just as the efficiency of firearms depends less upon the explosives and the missile they contain than on the judgment and accuracy of aim of the man who discharges them.

But to pursue further this train of thought would be to rehearse the themes I discussed before you and others upon a different occasion, and I will, therefore, conclude with a thought or two which, coming from the old to the young, may possibly bear some fruit in your minds hereafter.

I have somewhere met with an old saw—"Mean it when you're doing it." It is really only a version of the ancient precept: "What thy hand findeth to do, do it with all thy might." This counsel is full of wisdom. Whether the thing to be done be great or small, it should be done with such earnest attention as will insure its being done thoroughly. And as the sum of a man's life work is made up of qualities or units of various magnitudes, it may be compared to a Mosaic in which innumerable fragments of divers sizes, forms, and colors are combined to make a consummate picture, so does every one's life tend to harmonious perfection only in so far as its individual elements of thought, word, and deed are fitly framed together to produce a harmonious and consistent whole, free from ugly gaps, foul blotches and discordant colors, or disproportioned parts. Each, even the minutest, portion should harmonize with the rest and contribute to the unity of the picture.

We, all of us, more or less fail to compose a harmonious picture of our lives; fail, more or less, to obey the counsels of experience and wisdom, and we fritter our strength away in desultory and intermittent efforts among which we lose the habit of systematic labor directed to definite objects. The faculties of the mind, like the organs of the body, grow and are strengthened by appropriate use, but if allowed to remain idle become dull and sluggish, and may even undergo a sort of degeneration or atrophy. But a due variety and proportion of mental gymnastics tends to preserve them in harmony with one another and ready to co-operate in all the work they are fitted to perform.

The examples are many of naturalists, and mathematicians, and astronomers, and scientists in general, who have so warped and dwarfed their minds as no longer to have any relish for the beautiful in nature or art, or for those moral qualities by which human nature is raised higher than by all the dialects of the schools, the problems of mathematics, or even of the questions that concern organic life. The ancients bade us to "beware of the man of one book," not, perhaps, so much because he was apt to be supremely strong within the limited range of its special subject, and, therefore, to be avoided as its champion, but rather because its study would have tended to dwarf and weaken and emasculate those other faculties by means of which he could harmonize with his fellow-men, or oppose them in honorable conflict. No, the larger the range of one's knowledge and one's interests, at so many the more points will he touch his fellow-men in sympathy, and impart, as well as receive, the greater number of those ideas and sentiments that "make the whole world kin."

www.ingramcontent.com/pod-product-compliance
Lightning Source LLC
Chambersburg PA
CBHW050021230526
45470CB00003B/1076